TABLE OF CONTENT

It's an indisputable fact that time passes and the body changes. Your day-to-day health would be comparable to good weather and bad weather. Just as the sunny days are followed by short storms, health days are interspersed with colds, sniffles, pains and soreness, pimples and blisters. Your general health, however, would be more comparable to climate. Dependent on a number of factors, including genetics, luck, and your lifestyle, it has a greater and lasting impact on our lives. Every woman is unique, and the aging process will affect each of them in different ways. In general, to enjoy the best health possible at any age, you must understand the changes that can occur in your body. You will also need to take some periodic preventative exams and incorporate healthy habits into your life. Some of the factors that affect our health are out of our control, such as the medical history of our family.

At this point in your life, you are familiar with the foods you love and those you hate, but luckily your mind is still open enough to discover new foods on your plate. It may mean trying healthy and functional foods that you have never eaten. It is also very likely that it means eating less than before. In fact, as we age, the number of daily calories we need is lower; so you have to eat less. As our body's metabolism slows down as we age, cutting out calories can help us cut fat and prevent weight build-up. Given all our knowledge of how to live a healthy life and prevent disease, women do not have to worry about having supposedly reached the peak of their lives. Discover ways to live forty years in a dazzling way, taking the time to read.

- Ketones can be used as fuel for different organs, but they are mainly oriented towards the brain.
- Ketogenic diet excludes cheap foods such as cereals or industrial products and favors more expensive foods such as meat, fish or nuts. Its follow-up can lead to an increase in the budget devoted to food.
- In a balanced diet, lipids provide 35 to 40% of calories, carbohydrates 40 to 55% and proteins 10 to 20%.

- When the body is thus deprived of carbohydrates, fats become its main source of energy (whether from meals or from the reserves) and some of them are transformed into ketone bodies.
- It is advisable to drink at least 1.5 to 2 liters per day, to compensate for the low water intake of food (in general, high fat foods contain little water).
- Every week, book a few moments strictly for yourself. You can use your personal time to treat yourself to a treat, or to regain your well-being, relaxation or vitality.
- You can also make a list of things to do for the sole purpose of blocking the tasks you have already done.
- You may have to fight to find the time to exercise regularly. But every time you manage to do one more workout, as short as it is, your body will be a thousand times more grateful.
- The brain, which is a big consumer of glucose, can also use ketones when it needs them. It can therefore work perfectly even in the absence of carbohydrates in our diet.

Keto or ketogenic diet is a diet low in carbohydrates (fast and slow sugars), sufficient in protein and rich in lipids (fats). This mode of feeding can turn your body into a machine to burn fat! As a result, it is recognized for its beneficial effects on weight loss, but also on health, and on physical performance.

The term "keto" comes from ketones or ketone bodies. Ketones are molecules produced by the liver from fat as a source of energy. They are an alternative source of energy for the body no longer having carbohydrates as a source of energy. The brain, which is a big consumer of glucose, can also use ketones when it needs them. It will work perfectly in the absence of carbohydrates in your diet!

How it works?

In ketogenic nutrition, our diet consists generally of 5% of carbohydrates, 15 to 35% of proteins and 60 to 80% of lipids (in calorie intake). In comparison, the current diet called "balanced" contains about 50% of carbohydrates, 35% of lipids and 15% of proteins (50/35/15, it is a funny concept of balance anyway not?). Ketones are therefore produced when you eat very little carbohydrate (less than 20 g per day ideally), which has the effect of significantly reducing the insulin level and which, as a result, activates the oxidation (the "Burning") fats.

Therefore, the body that was working primarily on carbohydrates, will then draw all the energy necessary for its functioning in fat. Insulin is the hormone responsible for glucose treatment. Its role is to reduce the level of glucose in the blood. However, when it is produced, it has the unpleasant side effect of enabling fat storage. It will then block the consumption of what is already present in the body. In summary, when the insulin level goes down, the fat in stocks and food is more easily burned by the body.

In fact, when the body produces ketones, it is said that it is in ketosis. This state is natural. It is activated during a fast (deprivation of food). The ketogenic diet thus simulates this state (by lowering the insulin level) while continuing to offer taste pleasures with all the positive effects of fasting.

Why eat keto?

Speaking of benefits, keto is a great way to help with weight loss. But not only. Indeed, it allows, among other things, to increase its concentration, to improve its physical stamina, to have better health (tension, cholesterol, blood sugar), to slow the progression of type 2 diabetes, and is even recommended. for the treatment of epilepsy.

Keto is not the same for everyone

Ketogenic diet is safe for most of us. However, there are some exceptional cases in which we must make some adaptations:

- If you take a treatment for type 1 diabetes, this diet is beneficial to better regulate glucose in the blood but some precautions are to be expected.
- If you are taking a blood pressure treatment, this diet will allow you to reduce your blood pressure or even to make it go back to normal. It will however regularly monitor this and avoid consuming more salt, as recommended at the beginning of a keto diet.
- If you are breastfeeding it is possible to have a keto diet but in a more moderate way. You will lose weight during pregnancy while still providing good nutrients to your body and baby. For that, you will need to increase your carbohydrate quota to 50g per day instead of the recommended 20g daily.

All these details are given as an indication, but in these cases the best thing is to have a health professional accompany you!

What do we eat in keto?

The principle of the ketogenic diet is to consume as few carbohydrates as possible. In general, it is necessary to stay below 50 g per day but it is better to aim for less than 20g. The fewer carbs, the more the keto will be effective.

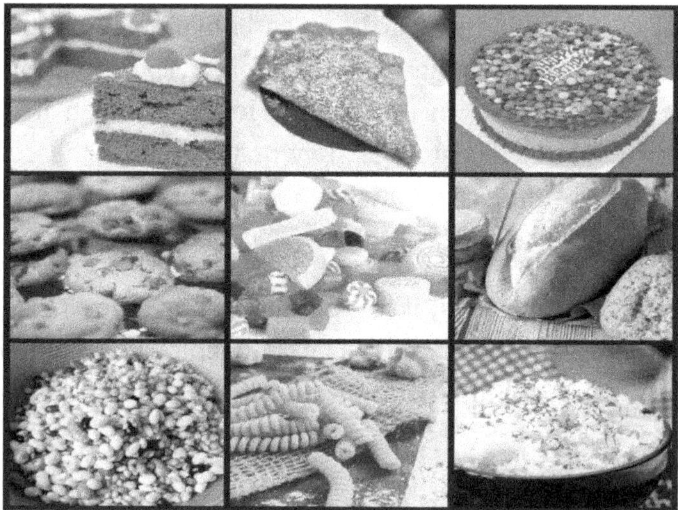

We have fun with:

- The good oils without hydrogenated fats (olive oil, walnut oil, flaxseed oil, coconut oil and avocado oil).
- Natural animal fats (duck fat, goose fat, lard and beef tallow).
- The seeds and fruit oilseeds (chia seeds, flax, walnuts and macadamia).

- The protein sources: red meat, poultry, fish (preferably fatty sardines, mackerel and salmon), eggs etc.
- Not to mention vegetables low in carbohydrates: cauliflower, zucchini, cabbage, spinach and broccoli.
- The dairy products (if not intolerant): go ahead cheerfully on butter, cheese, and cream.
- You can tolerate the lowest carb fruits such as avocados, berries or rhubarb.

We avoid:

- All sugars (white, red, agave syrup and honey).
- Products made from cereals (such as bread, pasta and rice).
- Foods rich in starch: potatoes, sweet potato etc.
- Legumes (lentils, red / white beans).
- Prepared dishes and sauces.
- Sweet products (such as cakes, sweets, jams).
- The very sweet fruits (bananas, apples, dates).

How to be in ketosis?

Several elements will allow us to enter ketosis and increase our production of ketones. Here are some rules to follow if you want to optimize this:

- Restrict carbohydrates: - Do not consume more than 20 g of carbohydrates per day (the fibers are not included). Consult the Ciqual table of TENSES for the macronutrients of foods.
- Have adequate protein intake: - It is important to consume what your body needs. The suggested amount is 1.2 to 2g per day (depending on your sport activity) and per kilogram of body. For example, for a person of 80 kg, 96 to 160g of protein will do.
- Eat fat: - Do not hesitate to consume fat to have this feeling of satisfaction. Unlike other diets that scare you, this one will make you feel good and you will not have that feeling of frustration. But do not force yourself either, there is no "quota" to reach. The right amount of fat is the one that makes you want.
- Avoid nibbling: - When the urge comes, ask yourself if you are really hungry or if it's just a habit. If you have eaten enough food, you will not need to nibble anymore.
- Try intermittent fasting (for example, eating for 8 hours and fasting for 16 hours a day).
- Playing sports: - This advice is not necessary to be in ketosis but it allows to accelerate the process and accelerate the weight loss.
- Get enough: - Lack of sleep and stress can increase glucose in the blood. This can slow the entry into ketosis and weight loss.

There are ways to accurately measure ketone levels in blood or urine using specific devices. However, we do not necessarily need this to know it. Some visible symptoms can identify if you are in ketosis:

- A feeling of dry mouth: We are often thirsty. You can also have a metallic taste in your mouth.
- A frequent urge to pee: This is due to the fact that we will drink more (see previous point) and ketone bodies that are evacuated in the urine. Moreover, when one consumes almost no more carbohydrates, one retains less water in one's body, so one goes more often to the toilets!
- Possibility to meet with a jackal breath but it will not happen necessarily, and it's temporary! The smell comes from the evacuation of ketonic bodies by the breath that is close to the smell of solvents.
- We are less hungry: Since the body gets used to using its fat reserves to function, some people feel less hungry. We are even able to do only one or two meals a day without difficulty.
- We feel more energy: After the first few days of adaptation to the keto, you can feel a boost of energy. This can result in a clearer mind, a more active brain, even a feeling of euphoria!

Ketogenic recipes for women at 40

The ketogenic diet is gaining popularity in recent years. It is an extremely low carb diet and very high in fat. We worked very hard to design a new menu that meets the criteria of this diet. To give you an overview of the recipes it could contain, here are some ketogenic recipes for women at 40.

1. **Asian vegetable and tempeh soup**

This recipe is vegetarian and ketogenic. The rice vermicelli from the original recipe are replaced here with konjac pasta that is free of carbohydrates.

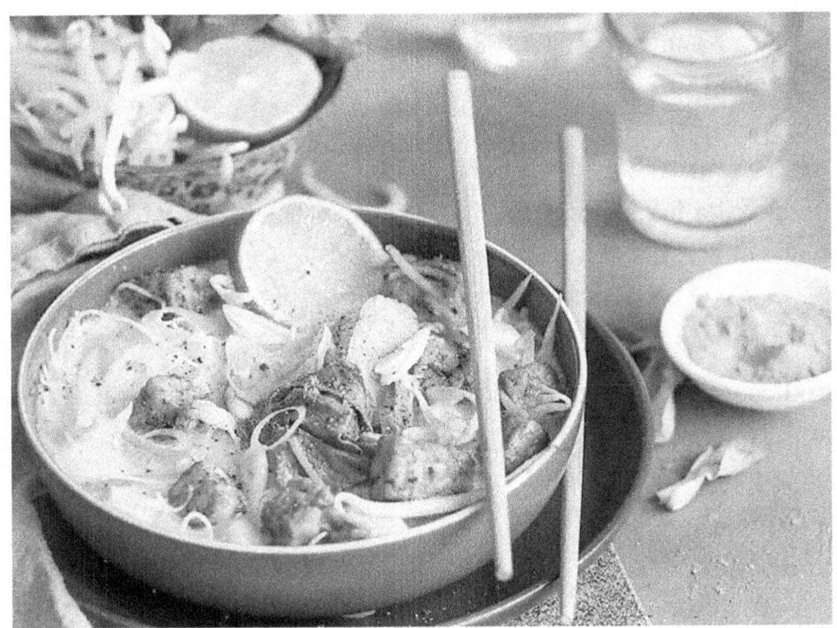

This recipe is: -

Without: Added sugar

Excellent source of: Calcium, Copper, Iron, Fibers, Folate, Magnesium, Manganese, Niacin, Phosphorus, Potassium, Vitamin A, Vitamin B2, Vitamin B6, Vitamin K, Zinc

Good source of: Vitamin B1, Vitamin C

Source of: Pantothenic acid, Omega-6, Selenium, Vitamin B12, Vitamin E

Low: Sodium

Ingredients

- 2 cups of vegetables soup 500 mL
- 1 cup   of water 250 mL
- 1/3 cup unsweetened coconut milk 85 mL
- 1/2 limes / limes, juice and zest 35 g
- 1 little bok choy 150 g
- 1/2 dried red peppers, finely chopped 0.2 g
- 200 g   shirataki noodles / konjac
- 4 teaspoons   coconut oil 18 g
- 240 g   tempeh, cut into cubes
- 1 teaspoon   curry / curry powder   3 g
- 1 pinch salt [optional] 0.2 g
- pepper to taste [optional]
- 1/2 carrots, finely grated 50 g
- 1/2 green onions / shallots, chopped
- 9 tablespoons bean sprouts 40 g

Method

- Rinse the noodles with plenty of water to eliminate the odor and drain well.
- In a saucepan, bring broth, water, coconut milk, zest and lime juice to a boil.
- Add the bok choy and red pepper.
- Reserve on a low heat.
- Meanwhile, heat a skillet over medium heat. Add noodles and cook for 2-3 minutes, stirring until all noodles are hot.
- Then move the noodles from the pan and set it aside.

Heat the oil over medium-high heat in the skillet. Y to jump cubes with tempeh curry. Jump until golden brown, about 5 min. Salt and pepper.

- Prepare the vegetables: Grate the carrots and finely slice the green onions.
- Spread in the bowls with the sprouts, noodles, tempeh cubes and cooking oil. Pour broth over.
- Serve.

2. Creamy rabbit with mustard

Rabbit meat is white, a little similar to chicken in taste and texture. It is found more and more commonly in supermarkets, because the rabbit combines a fine and delicate taste with very interesting nutritional qualities. Indeed, it is a meat rich in proteins, vitamins and minerals, and at the same time low fat and very digestible. Serve it with a classic ketogenic diet: cauliflower rice.

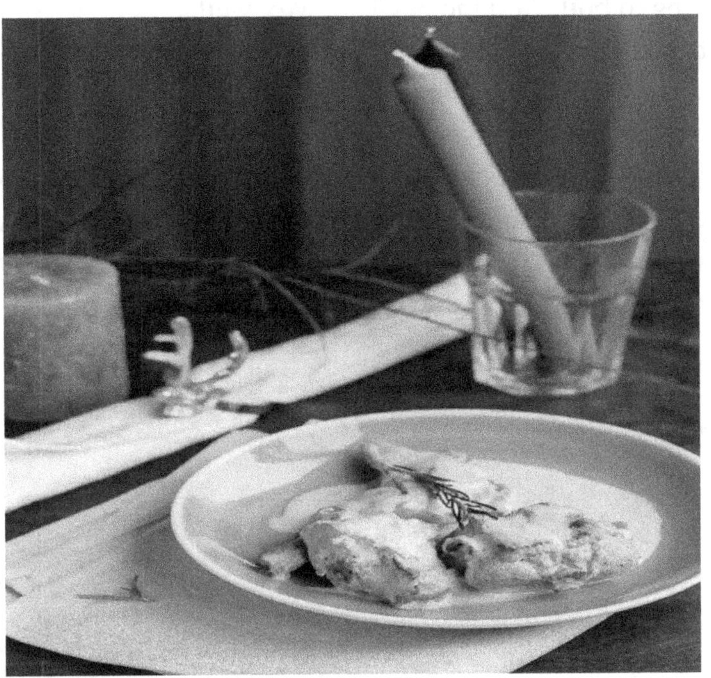

Ingredients

- 1 rabbit, cut into 6-8 pieces 1.4 kg
- 2 tablespoons olive oil 30 mL
- 1 pinch salt [optional] 0.2 g
- pepper to taste [optional]
- 1 onion, finely chopped 200 g
- 2 pods garlic, finely chopped
- 1/2 cup White wine 125 mL
- 1 cup   chicken broth 250 mL
- 2 bay leaves 0.4 g
- 1/4 cup whipping cream 35% 65 mL
- 3 tablespoons whole grain mustard

Method

- Before you start, heat the oven to 175 ° C / 350 ° F.
- In a casserole, brown the rabbit in oil over medium-high heat. Salt and pepper. Reserve the rabbit on a plate. Add onion and garlic and back until softened, about 3 minutes. Add the wine and scrape the bottom thoroughly. Put the rabbit back in the casserole. Add broth and bring to boil. Add the bay leaf. Mix well.
- Cover and bake for 2 hours, until meat is easily flaked with a fork.
- Meanwhile, in a small bowl, mix the cream and mustard. Book.
- Remove the oven from the oven. Remove the rabbit, bone it and reserve the flesh. Using a whisk, add the cream mixture to the cooking juices in the casserole. Heat 2-3 min on the stove. Return the rabbit meat to the casserole to warm and serve.

3. Brussel sprouts braised with bacon

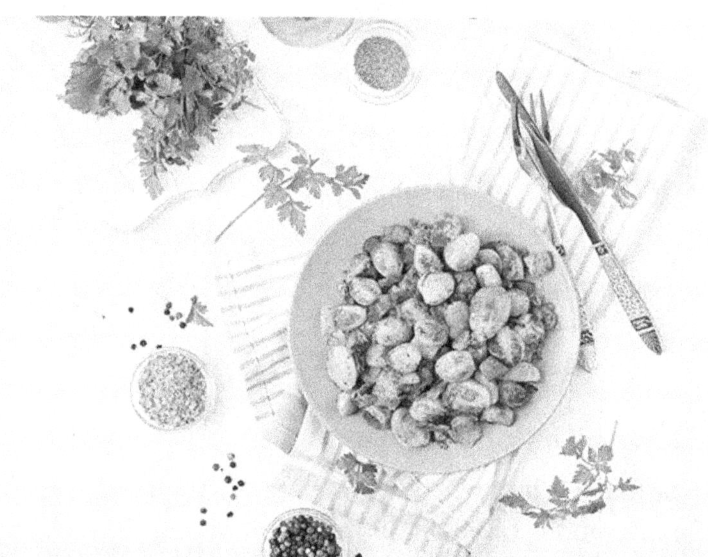

Green vegetables have their place on the ketogenic menu. In this recipe, Brussels sprouts become tender with a small smoky taste. Delicious!

This recipe is:

Health claims: Healthy heart

Excellent source of: Vitamin C, Vitamin K

Good source of: Folate, Vitamin A

Source of: Iron, Fibers, Magnesium, Manganese, Niacin, Phosphorus, Potassium, Selenium, Vitamin B1, Vitamin B2, Vitamin B6, Vitamin E

Low: Cholesterol, saturated fat

Without: Trans-fat, added sugar

Ingredients

- 2 slices bacon, chopped 40 g
- 2 tablespoons olive oil 30 mL
- 14 Brussels sprouts, cut in half or in four 360 g
- 1 cup   chicken broth 250 mL
- 2 teaspoons whole grain mustard 10 g
- 1 pinch salt [optional] 0.2 g
- pepper to taste [optional]

Method

- Chop the bacon and place in a non-stick pan. Fry until crisp, then set aside on a sheet of paper.
- Add oil and heat over medium heat. Add the cabbage and cook for 2 minutes stirring. Add broth and mustard, cover, and simmer until cabbage is tender, about 7 min. Discover, and continue to simmer until the liquid is evaporated, about 7 min.
- Put the bacon back in the skillet.
- Cook 1 min stirring.
- Salt and pepper.
- Serve.

4. Cauliflower popcorn

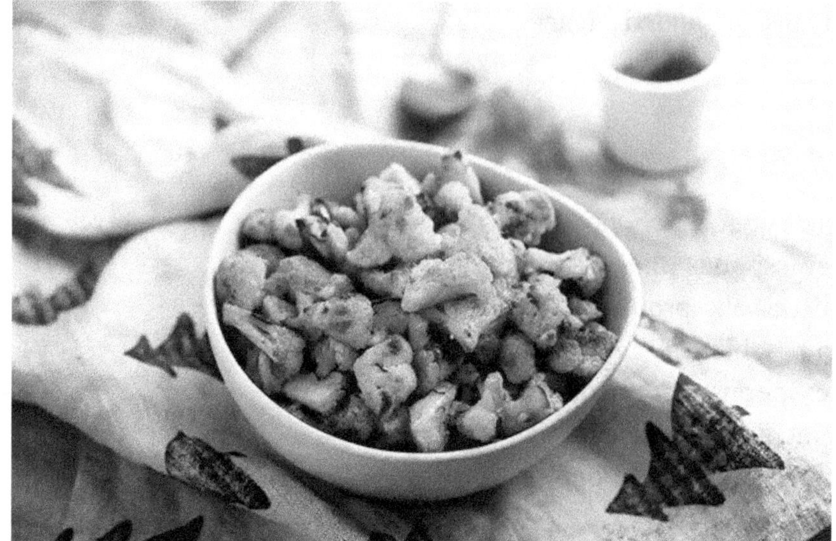

Cauliflower is a recurring food of the ketogenic diet because it is low in carbohydrates. And that's good, because we can eat it in all kinds of ways! Here, it is crunchy on the outside and tender inside in the form of popcorn.

This recipe is:

Health claims: Artery-healthy, Heart-healthy

Excellent source of: Folate, Vitamin C, Vitamin K

Source of: Pantothenic acid, Magnesium, Manganese, Potassium, Vitamin B6, Vitamin E

Low: Saturated fat, Sodium

Without: Cholesterol, Trans Fat, Added Sugar

Ingredients

- Parchment paper
- 1/3 cup olive oil 85 mL
- 1/4 cup wine vinegar 65 mL
- 1/4 teaspoon   paprika 0.4 g
- 1 pinch of cayenne pepper, or more, to taste [optional] 0.1 g
- 1/8 teaspoons salt [optional] 0.4 g
- 6 cups cauliflower, cut into bunches of uniform size 1 kg

Method

- Before you start, heat the oven to 230 ° C / 450 ° F. Line parchment paper with a large baking sheet.
- Pour the oil, vinegar, spices and salt into a large bowl. Mix everything well.
- Cut the cauliflower into small bouquets of uniform size, then put in the bowl with the vinaigrette. Toupin everything to coat vinaigrette bouquets. Spread these on the plate.
- Bake in center of oven until cauliflower is golden and tender but crisp, about 25-30 min. To brew from time to time.
- Serve hot or at room temperature.

5. Avocado egg casserole

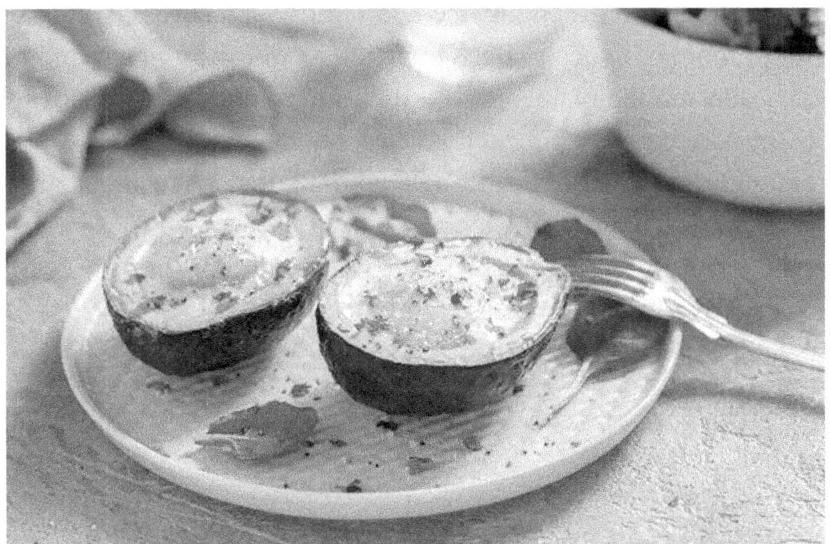

This recipe is easy to make and its presentation is pretty. It is perfect for a brunch or a light meal.

This recipe is:

Without: Added sugar

Excellent source of: Pantothenic acid, Fibers, Folate, Potassium, Selenium, Vitamin B12, Vitamin B2, Vitamin B6, Vitamin E, Vitamin K

Good source of: Copper, Iron, Magnesium, Niacin, Phosphorus, Vitamin A, Vitamin D, Zinc

Source of: Calcium, Manganese, Vitamin B1, Vitamin C

Low: Sodium

Ingredients

- Aluminium foil
- 2 lawyers 340 g
- 4 big caliber eggs
- 1 pinch salt [optional] 0.2 g
- pepper to taste [optional]
- 1 pinch Cayenne pepper 0.1 g
- 2 teaspoons fresh chives, finely chopped [optional] 2 g

Method

- Before you start, heat the oven to 220 ° C / 425 ° F. Cover baking sheet with foil.
- Slice the avocados in half lengthwise and remove the core. Using a spoon, remove about a spoonful or more of avocado flesh to create a hollow large enough to deposit an egg.
- Put the avocados on the plate and fold the foil around the avocados to prevent them from tipping over. Alternatively put each lawyer in a ramekin.
- Break one egg into each avocado half taking care not to break the yolk. Add salt and pepper to taste. Add a pinch of Cayenne.
- Place in the center of the oven and bake 15-18 min. Or until the whites have seared and the yolks are still a little runny.
- Garnish with chopped chives and serve.

6. "Fat bombs" cheesecake

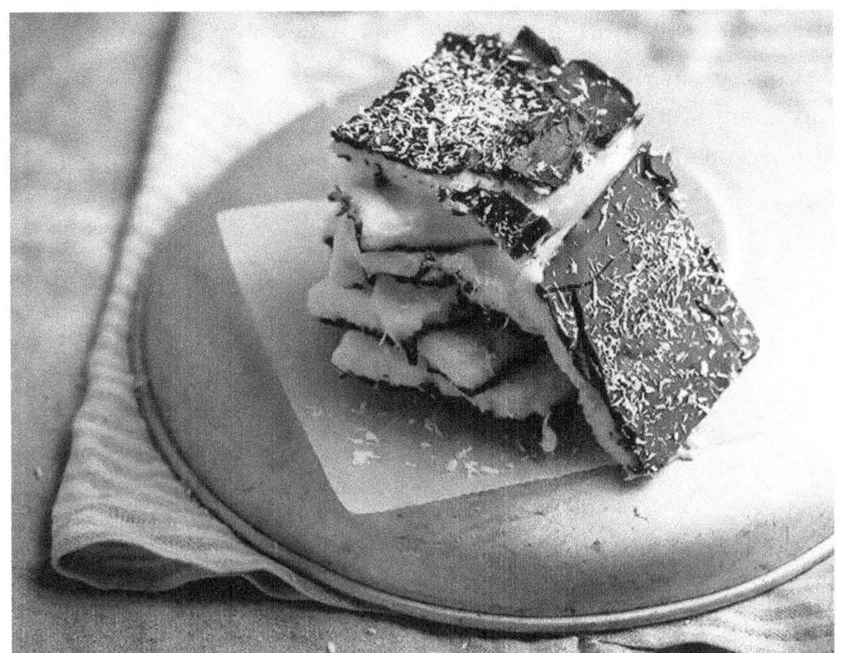

Fat bombs are used to meet lipid needs. For the sweet side, a small amount of stevia is used instead of sugar.

This recipe is:

Source of: Vitamin A

Low: Sodium

Ingredients

- parchment paper
- 3 1/2 tablespoons unsalted butter 50 g
- 4 tablespoons coconut oil 55 g
- 1 cup   cream cheese 150 g
- 8 drops liquid stevia [optional] 0.63 mL
- 1/2 lemons, for juice and zest 60 g
- 1 tablespoon   grated coconut (in filaments), unsweetened 5 g
- 1 teaspoon coconut oil, for chocolate 5 g
- 50 g bitter chocolate (black)

Method

- Prepare 12 small silicone molds or line up a 20x20 cm (8x8 ") square parchment paper pan to facilitate demolding.

- Melt the butter and coconut oil in the microwave in 15 sec intervals. Add cream cheese and mix well. Add drops of stevia (optional), the juice and zest of lemon and the grated coconut, mix. Spread the mixture in the mold.
- Melt chocolate and coconut oil in the microwave in 15-second intervals. Spread on the cream cheese mixture.
- Refrigerate until solid, about 1 hr.
- Unmould on a work surface and remove the paper. Cut into squares, to get 12 pieces.

7. Cheese and tomato pizza with cauliflower crust

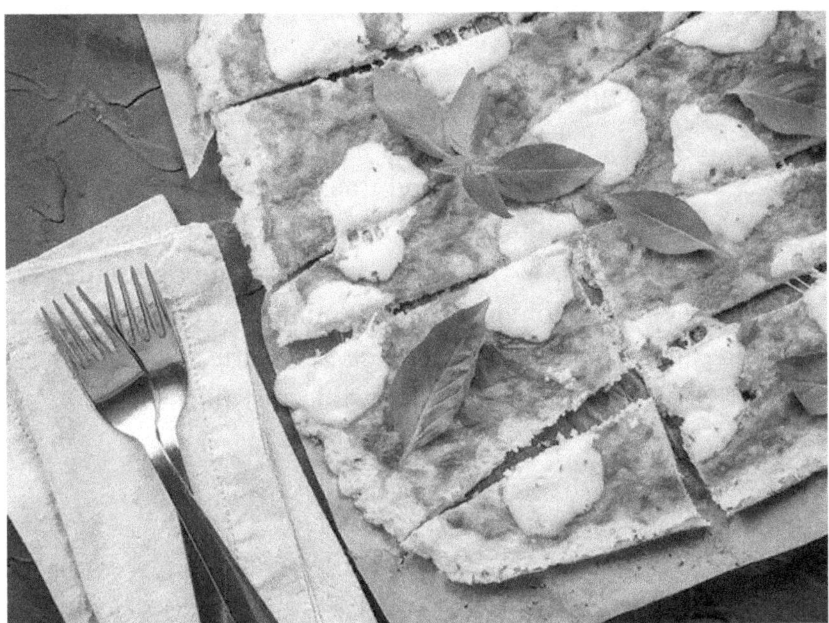

Fat bombs are used to meet lipid needs. For the sweet side, a small amount of stevia is used instead of sugar.

This recipe is:

Without: Added sugar

Excellent source of: Folate, Vitamin C, Vitamin K

Good source of: Pantothenic acid, Phosphorus, Potassium, Selenium, Vitamin B12, Vitamin B6

Source of: Calcium, Iron, Fibers, Magnesium, Manganese, Niacin, Vitamin A, Vitamin B1, Vitamin B2, Vitamin D, Vitamin E, Zinc.

Ingredients

- 3 cups cauliflower 500 g
- 1 clove garlic, minced
- 2 big caliber eggs
- 1/8 teaspoons salt 0.4 g
- 1/4 cup Mother's tomato sausage 65 mL
- 4 anchovy fillets 16 g
- 2 bocconcini / mozzarella 110 g
- pepper to taste [optional]

- 8 leaves fresh basil 4 g

Method

- Before you start, heat oven to 205 ° C / 400 ° F. Line parchment paper with a large baking sheet.
- Prepare the cauliflower and cut into bouquets and transfer to the cup of a food processor. Operate until cauliflower is finely chopped. Transfer to a large bowl.
- Add eggs, salt and minced garlic. Mix well and spread the mixture over the pizza crust.
- Bake in the center of the oven until golden, about 20 minutes. Remove the plate from the oven and add the tomato sauce, anchovies and cheese to the crust.
- Put back in the oven for 10-15 min. Garnish with basil leaves and serve.

Health tips for women after 40

No matter how old you are, maintaining a healthy weight is not easy. But from age 40, many factors can make your job even more difficult. Indeed, at the dawn of the forties, the hormones begin to make theirs. The metabolism slows down and changes begin to be felt. Perhaps this is the right time to make a small assessment. Do you want to take charge of your health and your body image? Getting back to balance requires first and foremost the adoption of healthy lifestyle habits.

1. Practice a physical activity

Our muscle mass continues to melt since our 20 years, in favor of the fat mass that settles gently. There is certainly no need to worry because in general, it is between 25 and 30% among women, and between 15 and 20% among men. It is essential for the proper functioning of vital organs, or to provide energy. The problem is that, as the needs fall, it is necessary to move so as not to store too much. And then, it's not insignificant, because who says muscle loss also says fewer calories burned.

Effective exercises for women 40 years and older

The arrival of the quarantine (and more!) Is a memorable moment even difficult! You already see that you do not have the same physical form as before. Rest assured! Even the most assiduous gym diva you admire will feel the effects! It's time to start doing effective exercises.

The physical changes that often occur between age 40 and 65 are:

- The loss of muscle tissue
- Bone density
- A decrease in metabolism which means that we burn fewer calories.
- If you do not change anything in your exercise program, you risk gaining weight instead of maintaining it.

Studies suggest that reducing the number of calories by consuming 80% of your usual daily consumption would help combat these changes. And a change in the way you exercise can help you burn calories more efficiently while toning up the areas to be fortified. Gennaro Ferra, a physical coach specializing in classes for the over 40 years, delivers 5 effective ways to exercise to make you feel better.

Stairs

To melt fat and develop your muscles, the exercises on the stairs are perfect. This helps to refine the silhouette while toning the legs during aerobics exercises. Take a sprint on the stairs (be careful though!) And jog down the stairs. If possible, alternate running up the stairs and jogging down the stairs for 25 to 30 minutes. You can add a bounce on one leg to make your glutes work more

The bike

If you suffer from muscular tension, knee problems, feet or back pain, cycling is an effective cardiovascular workout that will reduce tension in your muscles and joints. This activity will have beneficial effects on the lower body. If you are cycling outside, choose a course with climbs. This will require you to get up from the seat and sculpt your arms and upper body. Try to do a session of 45 minutes to 1 hour.

Swimming

It's time to remove the dust from your swim cap and go into the water! Swimming is a great sport for the chest and for the whole body. It increases heart rate, builds muscle strength and cardiovascular endurance and helps keep your heart and lungs healthy. Do a session of 35 to 45 minutes?

Kickboxing

This is an ideal session to burn calories while toning the body. For a complete workout, combine punches, kicks with a softer aerobics session. Kickboxing allows you to work the abdominals and burn up to 500 calories if you practice it for 45 minutes.

2. Control your portions

Since caloric needs are not the same at age 20 as at age 40, and, to complicate the task, the metabolism slows down and burns less energy, the first thing to do is to reduce the size of your portions, especially if you do not do any physical activity.

Advice

Use smaller plates: this will lessen your sense of deprivation.

3. Respect your satiety signals

We will not hide it, your days can quickly become an obstacle course: work that accumulates, difficult teenagers, activities to organize, house to manage, etc. It is not uncommon for you to eat your meal without thinking, worrying more about your obligations than what you eat.

Advice

Put your fork down regularly to give your body time to feel full. Also, it may be wise to leave the dishes away from your eyes; you will then have to get up to serve yourself again, which will allow you to evaluate if you are still hungry, or if you just succumb to greed!

4. Hydrate yourself

It is far from being a question of age; many of us do not hydrate ourselves enough. For some, this gesture is not part of a routine, a situation that gets worse as you get older, since the feeling of thirst tends to decrease with time. And should we really remember that water is essential to the proper functioning of the body, considering that the human body is largely composed of water? Drinking enough also helps eliminate waste and promotes digestion, circulation and cellular repair.

Advice

No need to do violence to you with large glasses of water since other liquids are just as good: flavored water, broths, juice, coffee or tea, you're spoiled for choice!

5. Limit your sugar and alcohol consumption

Several studies, including one conducted by the British Heart Foundation, have shown that it was sugar, not fat, that was primarily responsible for obesity. Worse, these calories are ingested without being burned and are then stored in adipose tissue, at the expense of muscle mass. Also be aware that alcohol, as well as soft drinks and some juices are extremely caloric and contain an unsuspected amount of sugar. One gram of alcohol equals 7 calories, while one gram of carbohydrate is only 4 calories.

Finally, alcohol is eliminated quickly, more than fat that will accumulate in the abdomen and promote diabetes, cardiovascular disease, hypertension or bad cholesterol.

Advice

Use smaller glasses that you will sip more gently.

6. Relax

Stress affects more than we think about our weight. When you are concerned, your insulin is stimulated and at the same time causes the accumulation of fat in the abdominal area.

Advice

Make an appointment with yourself. Book time slots that will only serve your well-being: a glass of wine while cooking your favorite dish, or an hour of massage!

7. Bet on proteins

But not just any! We favor foods rich in protein, but low in calories. This will allow you to be satiated longer and therefore less nibble. Betting on proteins by limiting lipids and carbohydrates will force the body to tap into its fat reserves to find energy.

Advice

Favor beef fillets or tournedos (no more than twice a week), white meats, fish such as tuna or cod, seafood and lean dairy products.

8. Increase your consumption of dairy products

At a rate of 3 or 4 servings a day, do not hesitate to vary the pleasures. Take the opportunity to slip into your snacks, which will have the advantage of being more satiating, because protein. Whether it's milk, yogurt or cheese, every opportunity is good to eat, especially when osteoporosis starts to be threatening.

Advice

What if you dip your fruit or vegetables in a vinaigrette or yogurt dip mixed with your favorite ingredients? It's time to give free rein to your imagination.

9. Do not neglect fruits and vegetables

They are filled with vitamins, antioxidants, minerals and fiber, essential to the proper functioning of intestinal transit and digestion. For information on the best fruits and vegetables for you, you can read this article: Top 10 fruits and vegetables. According to Canada's Food Guide, it is recommended to eat between 7 and 10 servings of fruits and vegetables daily, including at least one dark green vegetable and one orange vegetable.

Advice

Some nutritionists recommend a ratio of 2 or 3 vegetables for a fruit, the latter may be richer in sugars.

10. Limit your salt intake

Sodium is important for our body, especially because it allows the proper distribution of water in our body and the regulation of blood pressure, while participating in the proper functioning of muscles and heart, among others. Except that, consumed too much, it can have the opposite effect by increasing blood pressure, increasing the risk of cardiovascular problems or by promoting water retention.

Advice

Avoid as much as possible prepared meals purchased at the grocery store and pay attention to the nutritional information of these products. And above all, taste your dishes before adding a dose of salt unnecessarily.

The main transformations of the body at 40 years

Every time we move to another decade, be it 10, 20, 30 or 40 years, in our minds, it's as if we've just crossed another important stage of life. But why does the threshold of 40 years seem so different? Why do we feel that in our forties we have just reached the top of the hill and can only go down into the old age valley? To sum up the answer in one word and one: estrogen. In women, the shock of quarantine comes mainly from the fact that this decade corresponds to the decline of their fertility. It is at this age that many women enter the perimenopausal phase, the years that will lead to true menopause. Some women go into menopause very quickly in about 2 years, while others experience more discreet and obvious changes over the years, or even 10 years.

During perimenopause, estrogen levels fluctuate, triggering a change in menstruation - sometimes they are lighter, shorter, sometimes more intense or longer. The intervals between the rules may also change, and will tend to be different from those before. When ovulation becomes irregular, it is more difficult to become pregnant. While two-thirds of women over 40 have fertility problems, those who are pregnant also face a higher risk of complications (increased blood pressure or diabetes during pregnancy), miscarriage, birth defects, and low birth weight. These hormonal fluctuations can lead to menopausal symptoms, including hot flashes and sleep disturbances, with or without night sweats. Mood swings, irritability and depression may also occur, but they are more related to stress or lack of sleep than to hormonal fluctuations.

The loss of estrogen can cause a loss of vaginal lubrication, which can make sex difficult, sometimes painful, while exposing more women to infections of the vagina and urinary tract. There is also a link between estrogen loss and bone loss, hence the importance of supporting your bones with strength training and adequate calcium supplementation (1,000 mg daily). On the other hand, the lower the estrogen level, the higher the risk of cardiovascular disease, due to excessive consumption of bad cholesterol, decreased arterial elasticity and abdominal fat accumulation.

The abdominal fat - known colloquially as "belly" - may increase in women the risk of heart disease, diabetes and cancer. It is also a stubborn fat, because even with regular exercise, it can be difficult to control this part of your body and your overall weight. This can be explained by the fact that the woman's caloric needs change as she gets older, even if her level of physical activity does not change. The basal metabolism slowly slows down every 10 years, so it takes more effort to burn fat. Losing fat is not just a matter of aesthetics, nor are some other changes in appearance in a woman who is getting older. The signs of aging may become more visible as wrinkles, dry skin, sagging skin around the neck, wrinkles around the eyes and mouth. Hair and hair can whiten or gray and become finer.

In her forties, the woman can also observe a change of appearance of her breasts. Breasts consist of fatty tissue and do not contain muscles. It is an underlying network of connective tissues, called upper peripheral ligaments, and wearing a well-fitting bra, which support the breasts. As you get older, the ligaments relax, making the breasts flabby. When we enter midlife, we are also concerned about a whole host of other risk factors for our health. Osteoarthritis, a joint disease that usually affects the hips, knees, feet and spine tends to manifest itself in the forties and fifties, although it may occur at any age. The risk of breast, ovarian and uterine cancer also increases to 40 years, and becomes even higher, in the case of breast and uterine cancer, at the age of fifty.

The weakening of the pelvic muscles could contribute to urinary disorders such as incontinence. In some women, these disorders result from a condition called pelvic prolapse. Obese women or those who have had children are more likely to have pelvic prolapse. On the other hand, being overweight can increase the risk of uterine fibroids; these are non-cancerous tumors that develop in the years before menopause. Given all our knowledge of how to live a healthy life and prevent disease, women do not have to worry about having supposedly reached the peak of their lives. Discover ways to live forty years in a dazzling way, taking the time to read Your 40 years: health habits.

- Crunch your age: At this point in your life, you are familiar with the foods you love and those you hate, but luckily your mind is still open enough to discover new foods on your plate. It may mean trying healthy and functional foods that you have never eaten. It is also very likely that it means eating less than before. In fact, as we age, the number of daily calories we need is lower; so you have to eat less. As our body's metabolism slows down as we age, cutting out calories can help us cut fat and prevent weight build-up.

- Choose functional foods: Why should you choose? You can enjoy both by choosing the foods that appeal to your palate and by focusing on the best nutrients for quarantine. In this way, you will not have to worry about the number of milligrams or the number of micrograms of such vitamin or mineral. A balanced and varied diet, rich in fruits, vegetables, whole grains and low-fat protein sources, will probably allow you to meet the calcium and vitamin D needs to strengthen the bones, and the amount of fiber needed to preserve your heart and digestive health.

- Remember your magic numbers: While it's less stressful not to have to think of every specific true number of the recommended daily intake for each nutrient, it does not hurt to keep these values in mind - or stick to a sticker on the refrigerator. Here are some good facts to know about vitamins and nutritional values:

- Calcium and Vitamin D - Both of these play a big role in reducing bone loss that occurs during your 40s and 50s because of fluctuating estrogen levels and final declines. You must consume 1000 mg of calcium per day and 400 IU to 1000 IU per day of vitamin D.

- Lipids - Lipids should not exceed more than 30% of your daily calories. Also make sure that most of this 30% comes from good fats, that is, mono and polyunsaturated fats and omega 3 fatty acids found in fish, nuts and olive oil.

- Protein - Your protein should be 10% to 35% of your daily calorie intake.

- Fibers - The magic number is: 25 grams, which is equivalent to about 5 1/2 apples, but it's better to stick to your fiber by varying your food and eating beans, popcorn, raisins, a variety of vegetables and whole grain bread. In general, a healthy adult needs 21g to 38g of fiber a day.

- Be sure to be physically active. You may have to fight to find the time to exercise regularly. But every time you manage to do one more workout, as short as it is, your body will be a thousand times more grateful. Think of all the good that can bring you a new momentum of physical activity - sleep better, better manage your stress while keeping your cool, and enjoy a lot of energy both for work and for entertainment (from all the ways). Of course, if you alternate between aerobic and muscle building exercises, it will help you maintain a healthy weight, reduce the risk of many chronic diseases, and preserve and strengthen your bone mass. Rejuvenate your old worn habits by adopting a new approach. Replace your jogging session with a yoga party - or vice versa!

- Put your worries aside. If you suddenly find yourself between the tree and the bark having to take care of both your children and your elderly parents, you are part of the "sandwich generation". When we are faced with this situation, we risk very quickly not being able to manage our stress and our obligations. Finding time for yourself can be a real worry. Arrange to put your worries aside. Every week, book a few moments strictly for yourself. You can use your personal time to treat yourself to a treat, or to regain your well-being, relaxation or vitality. You can also make a list of things to do for the sole purpose of blocking the tasks you have already done.

- Let your beauty shine. Some signs of age reflect the joy of living: the famous crow's feet around the smiling eyes, or the small lines of expression of laughter. Others reveal the stress and experience of more difficult moments of life, such as the deep folds between the eyes or the frowns frowning with worry. Rather than yield to the temptations to hide these revelations of age - with a thick foundation, a paralyzing injection into the temples or even remodelling or lifting your face - find ways to shine your real beauty. Keep your skin supple by drinking lots of water and eating foods rich in antioxidants. Add antioxidant-rich skincare products that help restore skin that is marked by the sun or stress. Look for products with labels that say words like CoQ10 and Vitamins A, C, and E. Apply a moisturizer and use a regular exfoliator to get rid of dry, dull skin. Protect your skin from further sun exposure by applying a sunscreen moisturizer. If you feel that your skin needs even more help, ask your doctor about prescription medications that can reduce the appearance of brown spots, rough skin, or small wrinkles caused by skin lesions. skin. Protect your skin from further sun exposure by applying a sunscreen moisturizer. If you feel that your skin needs even more help, ask your doctor about prescription medications that can reduce the appearance of brown spots, rough skin, or small wrinkles caused by skin lesions. skin. Protect your skin from further sun exposure by applying a sunscreen moisturizer. If you feel that your skin needs even more help, ask your doctor about prescription medications that can reduce the appearance of brown spots, rough skin, or small wrinkles caused by skin lesions. skin.

The checklist

Review the checklist below and join the schedule of tests and exams that are recommended during your quarantine.

- Measuring Bone Density (Bone Densitometry): When you are over 40, do not worry too much about osteoporosis, unless, of course, you fall into certain specific risk categories. Taking certain medications may accelerate the loss of bone density, as may the presence of certain medical conditions. Talk to your doctor if you are concerned about osteoporosis, especially if your family is at risk.
- Diabetes Screening: If you are in your 40s, you may be at risk of developing type 2 diabetes. Your doctor may check for this risk by measuring your hemoglobin A1C (a blood test that tells you what your blood glucose level is) in the last 3 months) or your blood glucose level. The frequency of screening tests depends on the risk of diabetes that

you present. If you are overweight, your risk of diabetes will probably be higher and you should do this sooner or more often. Ask your doctor how often you need to be tested for diabetes.

- Blood pressure and cholesterol: You are not very exposed to high blood pressure or cholesterol, especially if you follow healthy habits for your heart such as regular exercise, healthy eating and not smoking. Whatever the reason for your medical consultation, you will be asked to roll up your sleeve for a blood pressure measurement. As for your cholesterol level, it needs to be checked every few years. However, if you enter certain risk groups, it is likely that your doctor will request this analysis more often or at a younger age. If you have diabetes, if your waistline is high or you smoke, your risk is higher.
- Pap test and pelvic exam: Since your 20 years, you are supposed to have a Pap test and a pelvic exam regularly, every 2 or 3 years. The Pap test can detect cancer of the cervix while the pelvic exam allows the health professional to examine the cervix and vagina, and determine the state of health of the cervix. 'uterus. Signs of infection may also be detected during this examination.
- Breast examination: Breast cancer is a very common cancer in women. Also, along with your Pap test and pelvic exam, your doctor could perform a breast exam. Ask if you need a clinical breast examination and, if so, how often. For your part, you should be familiar with the appearance and feel of your breasts when they are normal. If you enter the High Breast Cancer risk category, your doctor is likely to recommend that you have mammograms during your quarantine. Otherwise, mammography is recommended every 2 or 3 years between the ages of 50 and 74 (your doctor will advise you if you need to continue having a mammogram after 74 years).
- Skin examination: Skin cancer can occur in anyone, at any age. In addition to sun protection measures to reduce your risk, a comprehensive annual check-up by your doctor will identify new moles or spots, or those with changes in their appearance. You can perform a self-examination of the skin (or ask for the help of a partner). When you examine the spots or marks on your skin, here's what to look for (summary in 5 letters ABCDE):
    - A symmetry (non-rounded form)
    - B junk (outline with irregularities)
    - C-olour (color variation; difference from the other moles)
    - D-iameter (bigger than a pencil eraser)
    - É evolution (change in size, shape or color)
    - If anything seems unnatural or disturbing, talk to your doctor.
- Dental examination: make an appointment periodically with your dentist for examinations and preventive cleanings. The frequency of visits depends on the needs of each person, but in general, authorities in this area recommend at least one or two visits per year.

- Eye Exam: Even with a 20/20 vision, you should have an eye exam every 1 to 2 years. After all, the test is not just about the quality of your vision and the optometrist is looking for, for example, signs of glaucoma. If you have diabetes or high blood pressure, or vision problems are common in your family, the optometrist will inform you of the need for an eye exam more frequently.
- Vaccinations: Do you think vaccines are only for children? You may need a booster dose of some childhood vaccines; In addition, you can benefit from the protection offered by new vaccines against certain health problems that could pose a risk for you. Ask your doctor if any of the vaccines listed below would be appropriate for you:
  - Get vaccinated against measles, mumps and rubella (MMR) if you have never had this vaccine. The MMR vaccine would also be recommended if any of the following risk situations apply to you: working in health care, attending a college or university, and traveling to certain countries.
  - The vaccine against diphtheria, tetanus, and whooping cough (DTPa) is recommended for anyone whose last vaccine is more than 10 years old. Other groups that should receive the DTPa vaccine include people who work with babies, those who plan to become pregnant, and those who have had a contaminated wound (caused by a rusty nail, for example).
  - Every year, get a flu shot. This vaccination is particularly important in the presence of health problems that increase your risk of complications during an influenza.